Understanding Amlodipine Usage

Dr. Thomas Deriksen

Copyright © 2024 by Dr. Thomas Deriksen

All rights reserved.

Disclaimer

The data gave on this stage is to instructive and educational purposes as it were. It isn't expected as a substitute for proficient clinical counsel, conclusion, or treatment. Continuously look for the counsel of your doctor or other qualified wellbeing supplier with any inquiries you might have in regards to an ailment. Never ignore proficient clinical guidance or postpone in looking for it in light of something you have perused on this stage.

Table of Contents

Chapter one 5
Introduction to Amlodipine 5
chapter two 8
uses 8
chapter THREE 11
SIDE EFFECT 11
Chapter FOUR 15
INTERACTION 15
chapter five 19
PRECAUTION 19
Chapter six 23
DOSAGE 23
Chapter seven 28
FAQ 28

Chapter one

Introduction to Amlodipine

Amlodipine is a long-acting dihydropyridine calcium channel blocker primarily used to treat hypertension (high blood pressure) and angina (chest pain). It works by relaxing the blood vessels, allowing for easier blood flow, which effectively reduces blood pressure and relieves the heart's workload. Since its introduction in the late 1980s, amlodipine has become one of the most prescribed medications in its class worldwide.

History and Development

Developed by Pfizer, amlodipine was first approved for medical use in the United States in 1997. Its development was rooted in the need for effective and long-lasting medications to manage cardiovascular conditions. The compound's efficacy in lowering blood pressure and relieving angina made it a significant addition to the therapeutic options available to healthcare providers. Over the years, extensive research has validated its safety and effectiveness, leading to its widespread use.

Importance in Cardiovascular Medicine

Amlodipine plays a crucial role in the management of cardiovascular diseases. Hypertension is a leading risk factor for heart disease and stroke, affecting millions globally. By effectively controlling blood pressure, amlodipine helps prevent complications such as heart attack, kidney damage, and cardiovascular events. Additionally, its ability to manage angina symptoms enhances patients' quality of life, allowing them to engage in daily activities without discomfort.

Key Features

- **Mechanism of Action:** Amlodipine selectively inhibits calcium influx into vascular smooth muscle and cardiac muscle, promoting vasodilation and lowering systemic vascular resistance.
- **Dosing Convenience:** Amlodipine's long half-life enables once-daily dosing, improving patient adherence.

- **Safety Profile:** Generally well tolerated, with a favorable side effect profile compared to some other antihypertensive.

As a cornerstone in the treatment of hypertension and angina, amlodipine represents a significant advancement in cardiovascular therapy. Its efficacy, safety, and patient-friendly dosing make it an invaluable option for clinicians. In the following chapters, we will delve deeper into the mechanisms, uses, side effects, and future directions of amlodipine in clinical practice.

chapter two

uses

Indications and Uses of Amlodipine

Hypertension

Amlodipine is primarily indicated for the treatment of hypertension, both as immunotherapy and in combination with other antihypertensive agents. By lowering blood pressure, it helps reduce the risk of cardiovascular events such as stroke and heart attack. It is effective in various patient populations, including those with essential hypertension and those with hypertension secondary to renal disease.

Angina Pectoris

Amlodipine is also indicated for the management of chronic stable angina and vasospastic angina (Prinzmetal's angina). By dilating coronary arteries, amlodipine increases blood flow to the heart muscle, alleviating angina symptoms and improving exercise tolerance. Patients with stable angina benefit from amlodipine's long duration of action, which helps manage symptoms throughout the day.

Coronary Artery Disease

In patients with coronary artery disease (CAD), amlodipine can be used to help prevent angina attacks and reduce the need for other antinational medications. By improving blood flow and reducing cardiac workload, it plays a critical role in managing the symptoms of CAD and enhancing the quality of life for affected individuals.

Off-label Uses

While amlodipine is primarily approved for hypertension and angina, it may be used off-label for several conditions, including:

- **Heart Failure:** Amlodipine can help improve symptoms in certain patients with heart failure, particularly those who also have hypertension.
- **Diabetic Nephropathy:** Some studies suggest that amlodipine may benefit patients with diabetic kidney disease by reducing proteinuria and providing renal protection.

- **Migraine Prevention:** Although not widely recognized, some practitioners have used amlodipine off-label for preventing migraines, given its vascular effects.

Special Populations

Amlodipine can be safely used in various patient populations, including:

- **Elderly Patients:** Amlodipine's profile allows for effective blood pressure management in older adults, who may be more sensitive to blood pressure changes.
- **Patients with Comorbid Conditions:** Amlodipine is often chosen for patients with concurrent conditions such as diabetes, as it has neutral effects on glucose metabolism.

Amlodipine is a versatile medication with a range of uses beyond hypertension and angina. Its effectiveness in managing cardiovascular conditions makes it a key player in treatment regimens. As we move forward, understanding the dosing, administration, and side effects of amlodipine will further enhance its role in patient care.

chapter THREE

SIDE EFFECT

Side Effects and Risks of Amlodipine

Common Side Effects

Amlodipine is generally well tolerated, but some patients may experience side effects. Common side effects include:

- **Peripheral Edema:** Swelling of the ankles and feet is one of the most frequently reported side effects. This occurs due to vasodilation and fluid retention.
- **Dizziness or Lightheadedness:** Some patients may experience dizziness, particularly when standing up quickly, due to a drop in blood pressure.
- **Fatigue:** Amlodipine may cause general feelings of tiredness or weakness in some individuals.

- **Flushing:** Some patients may experience a sensation of warmth or redness, particularly in the face.

Less Common Side Effects

While less common, the following side effects can occur:

- **Palpitations:** Some patients may notice an irregular or rapid heartbeat.
- **Nausea or Abdominal Discomfort:** Gastrointestinal disturbances, though infrequent, can occur.
- **Rash or Itching:** Allergic reactions may manifest as skin rashes or itching.

Serious Adverse Reactions

Although serious side effects are rare, they can occur and require immediate medical attention:

- **Hypotension:** Amlodipine can lead to excessively low blood pressure, particularly if combined with other antihypertensive medications.

- **Angina or Myocardial Infarction:** Paradoxically, some patients may experience increased angina or even heart attacks, particularly during initiation or dose adjustment.
- **Severe Allergic Reactions:** Anaphylaxis, though very rare, may occur in susceptible individuals.

Risk Factors for Side Effects

Certain factors may increase the likelihood of experiencing side effects:

- **Elderly Patients:** Older adults may be more sensitive to the effects of amlodipine, particularly in terms of blood pressure changes.
- **Combination Therapy:** Using amlodipine with other antihypertensive medications can increase the risk of hypotension and related side effects.
- **Preexisting Conditions:** Patients with liver impairment or those who are dehydrated may experience heightened side effects.

Monitoring and Management

Healthcare providers should monitor patients for side effects, particularly during the initiation of therapy or when adjusting dosages. Key management strategies include:

- **Patient Education:** Informing patients about potential side effects and when to seek medical advice can help mitigate risks.
- **Dose Adjustment:** If significant side effects occur, adjusting the dosage or switching to an alternative medication may be necessary.
- **Regular Follow-up:** Routine check-ups can help monitor blood pressure and assess for any adverse reactions.

While amlodipine is a generally safe medication, awareness of potential side effects is crucial for effective patient management. By understanding the common and serious side effects associated with amlodipine, healthcare providers can enhance patient safety and ensure optimal therapeutic outcomes. In the following chapters, we will discuss drug interactions and patient management strategies to further support the safe use of amlodipine.

Chapter FOUR

INTERACTION

Drug Interactions with Amlodipine

Amlodipine can interact with various medications, which may affect its efficacy and safety. Understanding these interactions is crucial for optimizing treatment and minimizing adverse effects. This chapter explores common drug interactions, their implications, and management strategies.

Common Drug Interactions

Other Antihypertensive

- **ACE Inhibitors and ARBs:** Amlodipine is often used in combination with these agents. While they can enhance blood pressure control, there is an increased risk of hypotension, particularly during initiation or dose adjustments.
- **Diuretics:** Co-administration with diuretics can amplify the antihypertensive effect, requiring

careful monitoring of blood pressure to avoid excessive drops.

Calcium Channel Blockers

- **Other Calcium Channel Blockers:** Combining amlodipine with other calcium channel blockers (e.g., diltiazem or verapamil) can increase the risk of Bradycardia and hypotension. Caution is advised in such combinations.

Statins

- **Simvastatin:** Amlodipine can increase the plasma concentration of simvastatin, raising the risk of statin-related side effects, including muscle pain or rhabdomyolysis. It's often recommended to limit the simvastatin dose to 20 mg when used with amlodipine.

Serious Drug Interactions

Strong CYP3A4 Inhibitors

- **Ketoconazole, Itraconazole, and other strong CYP3A4 inhibitors:** These medications can significantly increase the levels of amlodipine in the bloodstream, enhancing the risk of hypotension and peripheral edema. Dose adjustments or alternative therapies may be necessary.

Grapefruit Juice

- **Grapefruit and its Juice:** Grapefruit can inhibit CYP3A4 enzymes, leading to increased amlodipine concentrations. Patients are usually advised to avoid grapefruit products while on amlodipine to prevent exaggerated effects.

Implications of Drug Interactions

Drug interactions may lead to altered efficacy of amlodipine or increased side effects. For example, combining amlodipine with certain antihypertensive can enhance blood pressure reduction but may also increase the risk of hypotension. Recognizing potential interactions helps healthcare providers make informed decisions about treatment regimens.

Management Strategies

Medication Review

Regular medication reviews are essential for identifying potential interactions, especially in patients taking multiple medications.

Patient Counseling

Educating patients about the importance of reporting all medications, including over-the-counter drugs and supplements, can help identify potential interactions early.

Monitoring

Routine monitoring of blood pressure and renal function is vital when initiating or adjusting therapy, especially in patients taking multiple medications.

Understanding drug interactions with amlodipine is essential for optimizing patient outcomes and minimizing risks. By recognizing potential interactions and implementing appropriate management strategies, healthcare providers can ensure safe and effective use of amlodipine in various therapeutic settings. In the next chapter, we will discuss patient management and counseling to enhance adherence and treatment success.

chapter five

PRECAUTION

Precautions for Amlodipine Use

While amlodipine is generally safe and effective, certain precautions must be considered to ensure optimal outcomes and minimize risks. This chapter outlines important precautions to take when prescribing amlodipine, focusing on specific populations, comorbidities, and other considerations.

Special Populations

Elderly Patients

Older adults may be more sensitive to the effects of amlodipine, including the risk of hypotension and peripheral edema. Close monitoring of blood pressure and renal function is essential, and dosage adjustments may be necessary.

Patients with Liver Impairment

Amlodipine is primarily metabolized in the liver. In patients with hepatic impairment, plasma concentrations may increase, necessitating caution and potential dose adjustments. Regular liver function tests may be warranted.

Pregnancy and Lactation

- **Pregnancy:** Amlodipine falls under Category C for pregnancy, meaning risk to the fetus cannot be ruled out. It should be used only if the potential benefit justifies the potential risk.
- **Lactation:** It is unknown if amlodipine is excreted in breast milk. Caution is advised, and alternatives may be considered based on individual circumstances.

Comorbid Conditions

Heart Failure

While amlodipine can be beneficial for certain heart failure patients, caution is needed, especially in those with significant left ventricular dysfunction. Monitoring for signs of worsening heart failure is critical.

Severe Aortic Stenosis

Patients with severe aortic stenosis may experience significant hypotension if treated with amlodipine.

Caution is advised, and alternative treatments may be preferred.

Diabetes Mellitus

Amlodipine has neutral effects on glucose metabolism; however, it's important to monitor blood sugar levels, especially when combined with other ant hyperglycemic agents.

Risk of Hypotension

Given its vasodilatory effects, amlodipine can cause hypotension, particularly when starting therapy or increasing the dose. Patients should be monitored for signs of low blood pressure, including dizziness, fainting, and weakness. Educating patients to rise slowly from sitting or lying positions can help prevent orthostatic hypotension.

Drug Interactions

As discussed in the previous chapter, certain drug interactions can increase the risk of adverse effects or reduce efficacy. A thorough medication review is essential before prescribing amlodipine to identify potential interactions.

Patient Counseling

Educating patients about potential side effects, the importance of adherence, and when to seek medical attention is crucial for safe amlodipine use. Patients should be informed about:

- The signs of hypotension (e.g., dizziness, fainting).
- The need to report any swelling in the legs or ankles.
- The importance of regular follow-up appointments to monitor blood pressure and kidney function.

Precautions surrounding the use of amlodipine are vital for ensuring patient safety and treatment effectiveness. By understanding the special considerations for various populations and comorbid conditions, healthcare providers can make informed decisions, optimize therapy, and enhance patient outcomes. In the next chapter, we will explore strategies for effective patient management and counseling to further support the use of amlodipine.

Chapter six

DOSAGE

Dosage and Administration of Amlodipine

Proper dosing of amlodipine is essential for maximizing therapeutic benefits while minimizing the risk of side effects. This chapter outlines the recommended dosages for various indications, considerations for special populations, and guidelines for dose adjustments.

Recommended Dosages

Hypertension

- **Initial Dose:** The typical starting dose for adults is **5 mg once daily**.
- **Maintenance Dose:** Depending on the patient's response, the dose can be increased to a maximum of **10 mg once daily**. It may take several weeks to determine the optimal dose for blood pressure control.

Angina Pectoris

- **Initial Dose:** For chronic stable angina, the initial dose is also **5 mg once daily**.
- **Maintenance Dose:** This can be increased to a maximum of **10 mg once daily**, based on patient tolerance and symptom control.

Special Populations

Elderly Patients

In elderly patients, particularly those over 65, the starting dose should be **2.5 mg to 5 mg once daily**. Due to increased sensitivity, careful titration is necessary to avoid hypotension.

Patients with Hepatic Impairment

For patients with mild to moderate liver impairment, the initial dose should be **2.5 mg once daily**. Dose adjustments may be needed based on individual response and tolerance.

Patients with Renal Impairment

Amlodipine can generally be used safely in patients with renal impairment, but monitoring is recommended. No dose adjustment is typically necessary, but caution is advised in patients with severe renal impairment.

Pediatric Use

Amlodipine is not typically indicated for children under 6 years of age. For children aged 6 to 17 years, the starting dose is usually **2.5 mg once daily**, with a maximum dose of **5 mg once daily**. Pediatric dosing should be determined based on weight and clinical response.

Administration Guidelines

- **Route of Administration:** Amlodipine is administered orally and can be taken with or without food.
- **Consistency:** Patients should be advised to take amlodipine at the same time each day to maintain steady blood levels.

Adjustments and Titration

- **Titration:** Dosage adjustments should be made based on therapeutic response and tolerability. Increments can be made every 1-2 weeks, allowing sufficient time to assess blood pressure response.

- **Combination Therapy:** When used in combination with other antihypertensive agents, amlodipine can enhance overall efficacy, but careful monitoring is necessary to avoid hypotension.

Understanding the appropriate dosages and administration guidelines for amlodipine is crucial for effective patient management. By tailoring the dosage to individual patient needs, healthcare providers can optimize treatment outcomes while minimizing risks. In the next chapter, we will discuss the side effects and risks associated with amlodipine use to further enhance patient safety.

Chapter seven

FAQ

What is amlodipine used for?

Amlodipine is primarily used to treat hypertension (high blood pressure) and angina (chest pain). It helps lower blood pressure and improves blood flow to the heart, making it effective for managing chronic stable angina and vasospastic angina.

How should I take amlodipine?

Amlodipine is taken orally, usually once daily. It can be taken with or without food. It's important to take it at the same time each day for the best results.

What should I do if I miss a dose?

If you miss a dose, take it as soon as you remember. If it's almost time for your next dose, skip the missed dose and continue with your regular schedule. Do not double up to make up for a missed dose.

What are the common side effects of amlodipine?

Common side effects include:

- Peripheral edema (swelling in the ankles and feet)
- Dizziness or lightheadedness
- Fatigue
- Flushing (warmth or redness in the face)

Are there any serious side effects I should be aware of?

Serious side effects are rare but can include:

- Severe hypotension (low blood pressure)
- Increased angina or myocardial infarction
- Allergic reactions (rash, itching, swelling)

If you experience severe symptoms or signs of an allergic reaction, seek medical attention immediately.

Can I take amlodipine with other medications?

Amlodipine can interact with certain medications, such as other antihypertensive, statins (like simvastatin), and strong CYP3A4 inhibitors (like ketoconazole). Always inform your healthcare provider about all medications you are taking to manage potential interactions.

Is amlodipine safe for elderly patients?

Yes, but elderly patients may be more sensitive to its effects. A lower starting dose is often recommended, and careful monitoring is essential to avoid hypotension.

Can I stop taking amlodipine suddenly?

It is not advisable to stop taking amlodipine abruptly without consulting your healthcare provider, as this can lead to a sudden increase in blood pressure or worsening angina. Always discuss any changes to your medication regimen with your doctor.

What should I do if I experience swelling in my legs?

Peripheral edema (swelling) is a common side effect. If it is bothersome or severe, consult your healthcare provider. They may adjust your dose or consider alternative treatments.

Can I take amlodipine during pregnancy or while breastfeeding?

Amlodipine is classified as Category C for pregnancy, meaning potential risks cannot be ruled out. Consult your healthcare provider if you are pregnant or plan to become pregnant. It is unclear if amlodipine is excreted in breast milk, so discuss options with your doctor if you are breastfeeding.

www.ingramcontent.com/pod-product-compliance
Lightning Source LLC
Chambersburg PA
CBHW070959220526
45471CB00007B/3105